Caring
Questions

Caring Questions

Sensitive and Fun Conversation Starters for Caregivers

Jennifer Antkowiak

x

PITTSBURGH

Caring Questions
Sensitive and Fun Conversation Starters for Caregivers

Copyright © 2010 by Jennifer Antkowiak

ISBN-13: 978-0-9800288-8-1
Library of Congress Control Number: 2009924740
CIP information available upon request

First Edition, 2010
St. Lynn's Press . POB 18680 . Pittsburgh, PA 15236
412.466.0790 . www.stlynnspress.com

Typesetting and cover design—Holly Wensel, Network Printing Services
Author photo—Becky Thurner/Thurner Photography
Editor—Abby Dees

Printed in the United States of America
on recycled paper ♻

This title and all of St. Lynn's Press books may be purchased for educational, business, or sales promotional use. For information please write:

Special Markets Department . St. Lynn's Press
POB 18680 . Pittsburgh, PA 15236

10 9 8 7 6 5 4 3 2 1

For all of you who struggle
to find just the right words
for those you care about:
My hope is that you realize
that your presence, your smile,
and your kind touch
speak volumes.

Table of Contents

Caring Questions

Introduction

❦

"Sometimes questions are more important than answers."

—Nancy Willard, *American poet and writer*

"Communicate, communicate, and then communicate some more."

—Bob Nelson, *public relations CEO*

*H*ow well do you really know the person you're caring for?

* Sure, she's your mom and you've known her your whole life, but what was her favorite toy when she was a kid?

* How did she feel about her first kiss?

* What did your dad do when he was young that he would've killed you for doing when you were the same age?

> → Was there any big sacrifice your father-in-law made for his family that you'd never heard about before?

The answers to these questions are precious pieces of your family history; they are the stuff human beings are made of. To get the answers, you have to ask the questions! Ya gotta communicate. The old-fashioned way. Face to face, words coming out of your mouth kind of stuff.

As a caregiver myself, I know that words are hard to find when there's been a bad diagnosis or a setback in treatment. This is scary and unfamiliar territory for most of us. Conversation can be tough to start when feelings of guilt, worry and fear are swirling around inside. If your loved one is dealing with depression or anxiety (which is quite normal during these life passages), you may feel shut out or like you just can't say anything right. Trying to talk with someone who doesn't want to let anyone in can be extremely frustrating.

Please don't let any of that stop you from trying (and succeeding) in gathering funny, sad, sweet, surprising snapshots of life. These can become family treasures – or they could just stay as thoughts you choose to keep close to your heart, as part of a new, private, deeper bond you are able to create with the person you are caring for.

Caregiving isn't easy, but I love to remind people that it comes with benefits. The opportunity to strengthen and deepen a relationship is one of the biggies. For some of you that will come easily. But, if you happen to be one of the many caregivers who struggle with anger or heartache, taking the opportunity to get to understand each other a little bit more can help heal old wounds. Tender caregiving certainly has the potential to be healing and hopeful – for both of you.

With this little book you're holding now, I want to help you maximize the moments you have with those you care about, so that you can enjoy the blessing of your time together for years to come.

How To Use *Caring Questions*

Keep this book handy! No more wasting time in waiting rooms or sickrooms watching silly TV shows or reading old magazines. Make the most of your minutes and ask some Caring Questions instead.

If you want to lighten things up, I've got conversation starters for that. If you're in a reflective mood, I've got something for that too. Skim through to find those kinds of questions that can be entrees to meaningful connection. If you have never really *talked* with the person you're caring for, here is a gentle and fun way to begin.

If you're starting to feel worried about not having much time left with your loved one and you want to ask important questions but don't know how, use *Caring Questions* to help you find the words you need.

Reach for this book when you're so tired you can't think straight. Grab it when you need some help bringing calm to a stressful time (even though you're feeling pretty stressed out yourself – I know so well how that goes). I think one of the best things about using this book is that it will take some of the pressure off and allow you to ask questions that might feel difficult to ask otherwise; if you need to, you can blame your question on the book!

Along with these questions, I've included some effective communication tips for you. I hope you will use them to start conversations that you and someone you care for will laugh about, cry about, and hold in your hearts for the rest of your lives.

I wrote *Caring Questions* with the idea that you and, if possible, the person you're caring for could take turns asking and answering the questions. I've left you some space throughout the book to jot down any details you want to make sure to remember. (Yes, I mean it – go ahead and write in the book. I'm the author. I checked with my publisher and editors and we all say it's OK.)

Celebrate and cherish your time together! By asking each other the questions in this book, you and your loved one will have a deeper understanding of each other. You'll have a deeper understanding of yourselves. I know, because I've seen it work in my own life.

Talking Tips:
Effective Communication for Caregivers

🍂

*W*hat's one thing you can do that will make your life as a family caregiver easier, guaranteed? Improve your communication skills.

Good communication is essential to providing safe and effective care. Whether you realize it or not, as a caregiver you are called on to be involved in extremely high level communications on a regular basis: with doctors, family members, home health care providers, insurance companies, and of course, with the person you're caring for. From delicate diplomacy with your loved one to explaining complicated medical issues to a new nurse, your skills as a communicator come into play every day. Anything you can do to hone those skills will make juggling all the issues that come with caregiving so much easier.

It's a given that you will find yourself in challenging

emotional situations. How can you stay centered and project ease and calm? How can you be the most effective? I want you to recognize how important just a few simple tips can be to maintaining your sense of wellbeing – and not letting stress overwhelm you as you communicate with your loved one. It starts with, literally, giving yourself a little breathing room.

Before you speak...breathe deeply for a moment

In my first book, *Take Care Tips*, I helped caregivers commit to making their own needs a priority too, by putting on the brakes, blocking out everything else going around them – if even for just a few seconds – and taking a nice deep, cleansing breath.

This isn't something we're used to. We do a lot of rushing around, and as a result, many of us have turned into "shallow breathers." We deprive ourselves of the powerful benefits of simply taking a good breath and getting oxygen flowing through our bodies and brains.

Taking just a few minutes to concentrate on your breathing will help jumpstart your communication skills – really. Pausing for a good deep breath in and out will help you relax and pull your thoughts together. If communication feels tense or difficult, another deep breath will help to keep you centered and focused.

Try this:

Drop your shoulders and take a slow, deep breath in.

Visualize filling every little part of your lungs with cleansing, oxygen-filled air.

Let it all out slowly. And then do this one or two more times.

How did that feel? I hope it gave you a positive feeling and a sense of calm.

Communicate with silence

While you're in this nice place, and before you utter even one word, here are some silent ways to strengthen your communication skills:

Focus – Pay attention to your body language. These are the messages you send to others by the way you hold your body. Are you looking at each other? How close are you to one another? How's your posture? Are you gesturing or touching each other as you interact?

Look the person right in the eyes. Position your body so that you are slightly leaning toward the person to show that you are engaged and focused. Doing those two things alone sends a strong message about how much the conversation means to you. There's no "right" way to use body language. Some people are more "touchy-feely" and others more formal. But pay attention to those unconscious messages you may be sending without meaning to. Try taking a chance with getting a little bit closer than you both are used to – a touch on the arm, a hug, a big sappy smile – it might go over better than you expected.

But there is definitely one thing that's a *no-no:* multitasking! Stop texting, folding laundry or going through paperwork, and focus only on the conversation.

Listen – When you really focus on what the other person is saying, you will of course be more able to respond in a thoughtful, meaningful way. Sharpening your listening skills will also help you be a better advocate for the person you're caring for. You will be able to move ahead with confidence that you are communicating their exact wishes to others in their circle of care. Listen critically so that you're sure you're hearing what the person is actually saying –

instead of, perhaps, what you want to hear.

Analyze – Watch the person you're talking with as they speak to you. Do their actions match their words? When we are scared, angry or worried, we sometimes say things we don't mean. Use your skills of analysis before you react. You may be able to pick up on a nervous expression or gesture that leads you to ask follow-up questions and get to the heart of what the person is *really* trying to say.

Now, let's talk

With all of that in mind, let's think about the verbal part of communication. Keep remembering that, as a caregiver, you are involved in high-level discussions. Part of your job is to take in detailed information that you and others in the circle of care will use to make important decisions. These are what I'll call *caring conversations*, and you probably have them every day. Make these caring conversations a priority. Here are some tips for success:

- Make sure you are speaking slowly and clearly. A nice, even pace allows you both to fully process the discussion and respond in the way you truly want to respond.

- Don't be afraid to ask questions, and then ask them again ... of the doctors, other medical staff, and the person you're caring for, to make sure that you know everything you need to know and that your information is accurate.

- Take notes during especially important conversations so that you can refer back for specific details when you need them. Date your notes, too, and give them a "headline" so you can easily find what you're looking for later (for example, *"Testing Option Update 12/2"*). Remind yourself that your job is to find a way to meet the needs of the person you're caring for, and that doing this in an organized, thoughtful way can help keep you grounded.

Special Communication Considerations for Caregivers

As I said earlier, it's easy to take communication for granted. I'll never forget how I felt when a hospice nurse told me that as my mother-in-law's health worsened, she might get so weak that she wouldn't be able to speak. The thought of not hearing her sweet voice, and the chance that with everything going on I might not remember some of her words, made me sick. I started journaling with her in an effort to maximize our minutes together and preserve some of her thoughts, hopes and stories. I wrote in the journal exactly the way she spoke – using her words, her grammar, her sentence structure. When I read that journal now, I can "hear" her talking as if she were here today.

Unfortunately, the progression of many diseases, including dementia, certain cancers and heart problems, can bring on a variety of barriers to basic communication.

The person you're caring for might have trouble finding the right words or forming sentences that make sense. Someone who's dealing with an illness may stop showing an interest in talking, or may be too weak to talk. Vision and hearing changes in the person you're caring for can, of course, bring about changes in communication, too. Although these situations certainly present challenges for quality communication, try to think of them only as obstacles. You can get around – or over, or through – these issues if you remember that, by definition, communication is the verbal or nonverbal exchange of messages.

Think of these circumstances as a call for you to grow into a better listener ... a better observer. By actively listening to your loved one with your ears and eyes, you'll be able to experience the benefits of effective communication.

It's not easy to see someone you love struggle to find a way to reach out to you. You can help the person you're caring for to communicate with you by blocking out distractions. Three things to remember:

Be Calm – This will in turn help to keep him or her calm.

Be Patient – Let your loved one know it's OK to be a little confused. Pay attention to nonverbal cues and if it looks like he or she wants some help, go ahead and jump in with some suggestions for what he or she is trying to express.

Be Positive – Focus on being helpful and productive. Dwell on the parts of the conversation that make sense, not on the parts that are confusing or frustrating. Resist the urge to challenge or correct your loved one during a conversation. Gentle reminders are beneficial and productive, if done in the spirit of being helpful.

The questions in this book are meant to get you both thinking about things you may not have thought about in a long time, or perhaps never thought about at all. The questions will spark not just answers, but *conversations* that will very likely become a much-loved part of your day. Start by asking the questions of the person you are caring for, but be ready to answer them yourself! Don't be surprised if your loved one grabs the book right out your hand and wants to know a little more about what makes *you* tick!

When you are truly communicating with someone, you are not just talking to them, you are *understanding* them.

Finding the Words

Let me quickly tell you a bit about my experience with being able to find the words I wanted – needed – to say in my caregiving journeys. I am a professional communicator. I took my college communications degree and put it to work in multimedia products. I was paid to investigate, report and present news stories for 17 years as a TV news anchor. And I've been blessed with many awards for my work.

Now, I research topics, interview experts and present information that families can use to make their lives easier on television and radio shows, newspapers, magazines and web sites.

I got into the business because I love *listening* to people. I love hearing their stories and asking questions to find out more. Being able to – being *trusted* to – share those stories in a public way feels like a natural extension of the communication process for me.

I bring this up to point out that the kind of communication that needs to happen during caregiving can be tough even for a professional. My reporter skills definitely clicked in and helped me to navigate a variety of caregiving experiences in my life, including caring for my mother-in-law who died of cancer. I kept detailed notes as I questioned doctors, spoke with surgeons, and carefully, critically listened to the oncologist when he told us that her scans showed aggressive cancer.

I sat with my mother-in-law on several occasions when it seemed there were no words. But I found words to ask her about what she wanted, and how I could help with her with this new part of her life. I found words to make sure she knew how much I loved her, and to reassure her that our children would know all about her.

There were plenty of tough times that called for just the right words: trying to help and manage the variety of emotions that other family members were feeling, trying to keep my head clear enough to absorb critical information about new medications that I'd be giving her, helping my mother-in-law express herself when she simply could not.

The experience was life changing. Intense verbal and non-verbal communication between the two of us increased and solidified an already incredibly strong bond. (So strong in fact, that I've felt, and continue to feel, her presence and support since she's been gone.)

Difficult times, scary times, confusing times make some people yell, and others fall silent. I hope these questions will help you find a happy middle ground so that you are able to use your time as a caregiver to create a powerful, valuable connection of your own. If you are only now just building a relationship that had been rocky before, let these questions help create a foundation for it.

Some of these caring questions are rooted in psychology – formed and included to help you to get in touch with and work through specific emotions. Others are just plain fun. All of them will help to take the relationship you have with the person you're caring for to a higher level.

Caring Questions

Firsts

Everyone's life is full of "firsts." What do you remember about these milestones in your own life?

$\mathcal{D}$o you remember your first kiss?

—⋅❧⋅—

$\mathcal{F}$irst great love?

—⋅❧⋅—

$\mathcal{F}$irst night together? *(only for the brave!)*

Do you remember your first big argument
with your "special person"?
What was it about?

—⋅&—

First heartbreak?

—⋅&—

First honor or award?

Do you remember your first car?

—⁊—

First time on a plane?

—⁊—

First home?

Do you remember your first pet?

First big letdown?

First big paycheck?

First big purchase?

Notes

Notes

Relationships

The people you are close with have a big impact on how you move through life. Take a few minutes to explore your relationships. By taking the time to ask and answer these kinds of questions, there's a good chance you'll discover something new about yourself, too.

If you had to pick three people in your life to help you win a million dollars by a) answering a math question, b) doing a physical challenge, and c) making people laugh ... which person would you pick for each?

How would you describe your role in your family?

Why do you think you're a good person to be in
a relationship with?

What was the best thing anyone ever did for you?

What was the best thing you ever did for someone?

What one thing would you change about a
relationship of yours?

⸎

Forgiveness isn't always easy. Have you ever
had a situation where it was challenging
to forgive someone?

⸎

What's one thing I do that drives you crazy?

Tell me about a special pet you had.

——— ❧ ———

What's the best family scandal you know about?
(Use your best judgment about whether this is appropriate
for the situation, and if you really want
to know the answer!)

——— ❧ ———

If you had to write one sentence to the people in
your life to say how you really feel about them,
what would it say?

Notes

Notes

⤳

_____

_____

_____

_____

_____

_____

_____

_____

Stress Busters

Stress associated with caring for a sick relative can cause serious health problems for the caregiver and affect the loved one as well. These questions can help cut through the stress by taking you to some simple pleasures and fond recollections.

If you could go anywhere in the world on vacation, where would you go? Who would you take with you? Which family vacation do you remember most?

— ❧ —

What activity makes you feel the most relaxed and why?

What's the best part of growing older?

—❧—

Do you have any tattoos, and where did you
get your first one?

—❧—

If you could have a maid or a chef, which
would you choose?

What's one movie or book that always makes you laugh?

How about singing one of your favorite songs?

What's one word that makes you feel calm?

What's one thing that I do that makes you smile?

Notes

～◎～

Strength from Above

Research shows that people who pray regularly are healthier than those who don't. You and your loved one may have different feelings and beliefs about spirituality. Go ahead and talk about it, respectfully, and learn about how you each understand the meaning of it all.

Do you believe in God? Why? Why not?

Do you believe that you were put you here for a purpose? What do you feel it is?

*C*an you name a time that you made a decision based on a gut feeling and it turned out to be very right?

---

*D*o you believe that prayer or meditation can help you through life's challenges? Can you name a time when prayer or meditation did help you?

---

*D*id you ever get what you think was a sign from "above"? Why do you think you got it and what did it mean to you?

*I*s there a special prayer that you say before you go to bed or first thing when you wake up?

—⋲●—

*H*ow do you feel when you are in a place of worship?

—⋲●—

*D*o you believe that our souls go somewhere after we die, or do we simply return to the elements?

—⋲●—

*H*as anything ever happened to make you lose faith or struggle to regain it?

$\mathcal{D}$id you ever learn anything from a holy person in your life that changed your way of thinking?

❧

$\mathcal{D}$id you ever get the uncontrollable giggles in church or temple? What was so funny?

❧

$\mathcal{W}$hat would you tell someone who is mad at God about a situation in their life?

❧

$\mathcal{I}$f you made up a prayer for your family, what would it be?

33

Notes

~⚬~

Notes

∽⊘∾

Around the Water Cooler

Our life at work feeds into our life at home. Many of us live large parts of our lives at the office. Use these questions to remember and share some of your work adventures.

*W*hat was your first job? How old were you? How much did you make?

——— ❧ ———

*W*hat was your favorite job and why? What would be your dream job?

$\mathcal{D}$id you have a work accomplishment that made you very proud?

Were you ever fired?

What was/is your favorite part about your job?

$\mathcal{D}$id you ever take anything from work that you weren't supposed to?

*W*hen did you know what career path you wanted to follow?

—❦—

*H*as there ever been anyone you especially looked up to at work? Someone you would consider a role model?

—❦—

*H*as there ever been anyone you just couldn't stand at work?

What advice would you give someone just starting out in a career?

⁓

How did/do you feel about leaving the house to go to work?

⁓

What's the best thing about coming home after work?

Notes

⌘

Notes

❧

_____

_____

_____

_____

_____

_____

_____

_____

Family Traditions

From putting out the Easter baskets, to Sunday dinners around Grandma's table, traditions are a cherished part of our lives. Traditions are like glue, holding families together. Passing down details of family celebrations is a wonderful gift for the generations to come.

*G*rowing up, what was your favorite family tradition?

——— ❧ ———

*W*hat was the worst part about one of your family traditions?

When you hear the phrase "family tradition," do feelings of stress or joy fill you first?

———

What tradition were you/are you most eager to enjoy with your own family?

———

Is there a family tradition that stopped when a loved one passed away, and that you miss? Which one tradition would you most like to be passed down through the generations in your family?

*W*hat family tradition do you think made your
parents nuts?

❧

*H*as there ever been a tradition you wanted to share
with all of your friends?

❧

*D*o you feel you learned enough about where your
family traditions came from?

❧

*W*hat does your cultural heritage mean to you?

Notes

~⊘~

Notes

Notes

$\sim$

Our World

Our views of the world around us give good insight into who we really are. Chances are, the conversations you start with some of these questions will make you laugh. Others might make your blood boil! Respect each other's opinions, but allow yourselves to share how you really feel about these issues, and prepare for some possible surprises!

Do you vote? Who did you vote for in the last election?

Did you ever switch political parties?

How do you feel about using domestic money and resources to help people in other countries?

—⋙—

What is one of the things you've learned about our world that surprised you the most?

—⋙—

What bugs you most about people who have other political opinions?

What is one of the things you love most about
our country?

What is one of the things that frustrates you
the most about our country?

Where have you not yet gone that you would
like to visit?

What animal would you hate to see become endangered or extinct?

What is the biggest challenge of our time?

What is the prettiest natural site you've ever seen?

$\mathcal{I}$f you were able to be a scientist and travel anywhere to conduct research on anything at all, where would you go and what would you study?

$\mathcal{W}$hat other language would you love to learn?

$\mathcal{W}$hat other country, if any, would you like to live in?

Notes

~⚬~

Feelings

Dig deep. Let yourself think about and express your feelings. You might surprise yourself with your answers! Exposing your true feelings may be uncomfortable sometimes, but it's worth it. Give yourself a moment to take a calming, deep breath. And remember, honest and gentle sharing is a surefire way to create or strengthen a relationship.

When do you feel happiest?

—❧—

What makes you angry?

*W*hen have you felt the most jealousy?

*W*hat makes you sad?

*W*hen do you feel the most scared?

*W*hat makes you feel overwhelmed?

—⁓&—

*W*hen in your life have you felt on top of the world?

—⁓&—

*W*hat makes you feel silly?

—⁓&—

*W*hat's the most embarrassing thing that ever
happened to you?

What, whenever you think about it, fills you with the greatest feelings of love?

When do you feel annoyed?

What's the one thing you feel most days that you wish you could scream about?

When do you feel the most at peace?

Notes

✑

_____

_____

_____

_____

_____

_____

_____

_____

_____

Notes

Dare to Dream

Daydream a little! Be uplifted thinking about how you'd change the world if there were no time, health or money issues.

If you had a magic wand, what would you change about your house? Yourself? The world?

❧

If you could do one thing over again, knowing what you know now, what would it be?

If you had a spare hour/month/year, what would you do?

—❦—

What new skill would you love to learn?

—❦—

What daredevil type of activity would you like to try?

*W*ho do you wish you could do a perfect impersonation of? Let's hear your best attempt!

---

*I*f you could find a long-lost friend or relative, who would you want to track down?

---

*I*f you were able to change some discipline you dished out, what would you change and why?

Notes

School Days

The friends, the teachers, the fun, the horrible hair-dos!
Stroll on back to your school days.

$\mathcal{D}$id you ever get into trouble at school?
For what?

———— ❧ ————

$\mathcal{W}$ere there any fads that you fell into, big-time?

———— ❧ ————

$\mathcal{W}$hat did you and your friends do at recess?

*W*hat was your most and least favorite class?

—◦—

*W*ho was your favorite/least favorite teacher?
Why?

—◦—

*W*hat do you remember most about getting up
and getting ready for school?

What's one thing you didn't learn in school
but wish you had?

What was your favorite school lunch or your
favorite thing to trade for?

What was your favorite school activity?

Were you in any "group" of kids at school?
Were you a nerd or a cool kid?

Did you ever tease or bully anyone? Did anyone
tease or bully you?

—❧—

If you could go back to school again what would
you do differently?

—❧—

Did you ever break the rules and *not* get caught?

Notes

_____

_____

_____

_____

_____

_____

_____

_____

Notes

Hopes, Fears and Wishes

Use these questions during a quiet time together, when you both are relaxed and feel like you have the time to really reflect on these ideas. They are emotional, important conversations. During this time, it's especially good to have a pen or pencil handy to jot down notes.

How do you hope that your family and friends remember you?

—⋙—

What do you wish for your children/grandchildren?

What special words, songs or anything else would you like at your funeral?

If you could make sure that people remembered you at a particular time in your life, when would that be?

What are you afraid of?

*W*hat's one thing you lived through/experienced that
you hope no one in your family ever has to?

—ဆ—

*W*hat's one thing you got to experience that you
hope everyone you love gets to?

—ဆ—

*A*ny regrets?

Notes

~~

Notes

∽∘∾

Notes

_____

_____

_____

_____

_____

_____

_____

_____

The Best of Times, the Worst of Times

Feelings can change quite a bit over the course of a lifetime. Something you once thought of as your ultimate high or most miserable low, might not seem like such a big deal now. Discussing them now may help to re-evaluate priorities. Take some time to identify your own personal peaks and valleys.

What was the best thing you ever taught me?

What do you think was the best time we had together?

What was the worst meal you've ever eaten?

—⁊❧—

What was the best thing you ever celebrated?

—⁊❧—

What was the first time you ever lost a loved one?

$\mathcal{W}$hat would be the worst thing for someone
to take from you?

—⁂—

$\mathcal{W}$hat would be the best thing for someone
to give you?

—⁂—

$\mathcal{W}$hat was the worst gift you ever received?

What is your best advice for newlyweds?

What is your best advice for new parents?

Looking back, what's the best and worst thing about being young?

If there were one memory you could hold in your heart during the rough times, what would it be?

Notes

~⊙~

Notes

Growing Up

It's easy to forget that we were all kids once, each of us experiencing the world through fresh eyes and brand new, tender hearts. How have you changed and in what ways are you still a little kid deep inside? Go back in time and explore the good old days! (And maybe the not-so-great days, too...)

What children's story do you remember fondly?

———

What kind of odd jobs did you do as a kid to earn some extra spending money?

How did you get "the talk" from your parents?

—

Do you remember your first friend who was a different race than you? What was that like for you? For your family?

—

How did you get along with your parents? Your siblings?

—

How did your parents react when you got in trouble or misbehaved? What were typical punishments?

Did you ever get caught drinking underage?

Ⓒ

What's one thing you wish your parents had
done differently?

Ⓒ

Who was your favorite relative or family friend
to go visit as a child?

$\mathcal{D}$id you ever break any bones when you
were young?

Were you a happy kid?

Were you aware that your family was poor, or rich,
or something in the middle? How did that feel?

Where was your favorite place to go to be alone
when you were young?

*W*hat was your least favorite chore when
you were a child?

—❧—

*W*ho was the "black sheep" in your family?
(Careful…it could be you!)

—❧—

*D*id you ever meet a famous person when
you were young?

*W*hat was it like growing up when you did?
(Vietnam, World War II, the 50's, etc.)

—⊰❧—

*D*id you ever get caught kissing a girl/boy when
you were young?

—⊰❧—

*W*hat was your favorite toy?

Notes

_____

_____

_____

_____

_____

_____

_____

_____

_____

Notes

~∞~

Just for Laughs

They say laughter is the best medicine, right?
So, what's funny to you?

Who is your favorite comedian?

—❦—

Have you ever played a practical joke on someone?

—❦—

What's your favorite knock-knock joke?

What usually works to cheer you up?

⟶ ❧ ⟵

They say "Kids say the darndest things." Do you remember something a child did or said that really made you laugh?

⟶ ❧ ⟵

What makes you laugh out loud just thinking about it?

*W*hat makes you blush?

—⁓—

*D*id you ever do something really stupid at a party?

—⁓—

*D*o you remember a time when you laughed at something that you knew you shouldn't have been laughing at but couldn't help it?

Notes

∽Ꙩ∼

_____

_____

_____

_____

_____

_____

_____

_____

_____

Being a Grownup

*Responsible, on your own, and totally in control …
right? Being a grown-up isn't all it's cracked up to be
sometimes. These questions will get you thinking about
an important transition time in your life.*

$\mathcal{W}$here did you go on your first real date?

—✦—

$\mathcal{W}$here was the first place you lived after moving
out of your parents' house?

How did it feel to be away from home?

Were you ever arrested for anything ... or should you have been?

When was the first time you disagreed with your parents politically?

What was your marriage proposal like?

—❧—

Do you remember how old you were and where you smoked your first cigarette? Or tried something stronger?

—❧—

What's one thing that you really wanted to buy but couldn't afford?

What was one of your typical bachelor/
bachelorette meals?

⟶

Did you ever get a black eye? Give one?

⟶

What was your favorite junk food?

⟶

Do you remember the first big thing you
accomplished by yourself – without your
parents' help?

Notes

~⚬~

Notes

Things that Matter

*Sometimes a song is just a song; other times, it takes
you back to a special place in time. Think about some
of the things that really mattered to you in the past or
still matter to you today.*

*W*as there a book you read that really had
an impact on you?

—⁓—

*H*as your own writing brought you a deeper
understanding of yourself? Of life?

Have you ever made anything with your hands
that you were really proud of?

—🐝—

Do you like to sing or dance?

—🐝—

Did you ever play an instrument? How much
a part of your life has it been?

—🐝—

Did your parents approve of your music?

*A*re there songs you remember from important
times in your life?

—❧—

*W*hat television show do you remember enjoying
with your family?

—❧—

*D*o you remember your first drive-in movie?

*I*s there a special scent that makes you feel wonderful? Brings back a memory?

―≈―

*W*hat sports team win do you remember the most?

―≈―

*D*o you remember seeing a special concert or show?

*A*re there any entertainers, authors or athletes
that you miss?

*W*ere there any styles or trends that you really
connected with or felt really defined you?

*W*hat's your favorite guilty pleasure?

Notes

Notes

_____

_____

_____

_____

_____

_____

_____

_____

_____

Notes

My Wish for You

One of the many blessings of caregiving is that the journey opens up opportunities for deeper, more meaningful conversations. By being conscious of those opportunities and not taking communication for granted, we are able to dramatically improve the quality of life for the person we are caring for, as well as for ourselves and our families.

Sure, there will always be those times when it is difficult to communicate – when there is increased stress from emotionally super-charged circumstances. That is 100% normal. It requires patience and skill to breathe through and work through those feelings and be able to talk about them. Use your love to fuel the process. Plow through the difficult times. Allow for and get comfortable with silence. It has its place in the process, too. And remember, we are constantly communicating – sometimes most powerfully when there are no words. Pay attention to expressions and gestures, to be able to absorb the total message and fully appreciate the gifts of caring conversations. Medical research suggests that hearing is the last sense to go. If your loved one is in the end-of-life times, know that using caring communication will create precious memories that will live on with you and your family.

A personal note:

While I was writing *Caring Questions*, my family and I were taking care of my dear father-in-law in our home. The experience greatly reinforced my feelings about the importance of communication for caregivers. Opening my eyes, ears and heart allowed me to fully appreciate hearing Pap telling my children how much he loves them and will always be watching out for them ... listening to him laugh as he told us stories from his childhood ... looking into his eyes and feeling his gratitude as he told us all his prayers had been answered and he was going to go happy because we were "sending him happy."

Pap passed away just before this book was finished. In the last week of his life, he slipped back and forth between this world and another. Pap was not responsive when I held his hand, told him I loved him and I would miss him, thanked him for everything he had given us, and told him it was now time for him to go. I needed to leave his room to check on some noise I heard from the kids, and when I went back not even two minutes later, I discovered that Pap had gone.

I will always be grateful for the time we had together in Pap's last days, and grateful that we didn't waste a precious moment of it.

That kind of communication – leaving nothing unsaid that needs to be said, and finding ways to deepen our connection with our loved ones – is what I wish for you with all my heart.

Acknowledgments

Organizing passion into a nice, neat little package takes a team, and I am grateful for the talented people who helped put this book in your hands:

My husband Joe and our kids: Thank you for your constant support and inspiration. You are my reasons for everything. I love you. My step-daughter Bethany: a daughter, loving cheerleader, and quite the business woman. Thank you for fearlessly defending time for me to devote to this project. My sisters who love and support me always. I feel it, and I appreciate it. My grandmothers: One here, one in a better place...both my role models for strong, loving, caring women. My Dad: Your quiet voice of strength and reason pops into my head and makes me smile. Thank you for helping me to keep my head screwed on straight. My Mom and MeMa: I feel you both with me always. I know you are working magic to help me on this mission. Stay with me!

My dear friend Gina and her family (my adopted family) who scooped up a blonde polish girl and her family and care for us like your own. Maybe the fact that I married an Italian helps! Thank you.

My St. Lynn's Press Family – Paul, Cathy, Abby and Holly: We've shared laughter and tears as well as edits and designs and layouts, and it's wonderful. I love being on your team.

Pap: You began this project with me, and I know you are watching from above as it is released. Our caring conversations touched my heart. Thank you for letting me into yours.

God: I thank You every day for everything. In this case, I want to specifically thank You for putting this book into my head at exactly the time that my head needed something else! You really have that timing thing down, don't You?

About the Author

❧

Jennifer Antkowiak knows about caregiving. She's a wife, mother of five, and step-mother to one. She was a caregiver during the end-of-life journeys of her mother, her mother-in-law, and most recently her father-in-law (who died while this book was being written). These varied and deep experiences have fueled Jennifer's passionate mission to help the world's caregivers.

Coming from a long career as an award-winning newscaster, Jennifer now provides multimedia messages and tools to help people keep themselves and those they love happy and healthy. Her earlier book, *Take Care Tips*, gives self-care strategies for caregivers.

You can find out more about the jennifer Cares mission, get a variety of helpful articles and resources, talk with Jennifer and other caregivers and be a welcome part of our community of caring, at:

www.jenniferCares.com.

Also available:

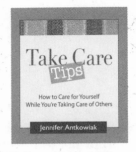

Take Care Tips:
How to Care for Yourself While You're Taking Care of Others

By Jennifer Antkowiak

In **Take Care Tips**, Jennifer Antkowiak offers *101 guilt-free ten-minute tips to help caregivers feel more hope, energy and joy.* With warmth and understanding, Jennifer shares her personal caregiving experience and presents authoritative information from medical doctors, psychologists, fitness pros, nutritionists, and other experts. The result is a book of easy-to-accomplish action plans that take little time and lead to renewed energy and wellbeing.

Take Care Tips can be purchased at bookstores nationwide and online booksellers. ($14.95, St. Lynn's Press)

www.takecaretips.com